SMK

Sumi Mathew
4483879 .
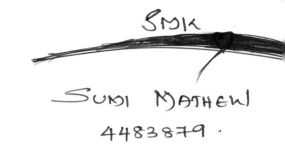

Essentials in Hospice and Palliative Care:
A PRACTICAL RESOURCE FOR EVERY NURSE

LEARNING ACTIVITIES

Katherine Murray
RN, BSN, MA, CHPCN(C)

Life and Death Matters
Victoria, BC

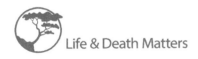

Life & Death Matters

www.lifeanddeathmatters.ca

Published by Life and Death Matters, Victoria, BC, Canada
www.lifeanddeathmatters.ca

Illustrations by Joanne Thomson
Editing by Ann-Marie Gilbert
Design by Greg Glover

ISBN 978-1-926923-13-0

Disclaimer
This book is intended only as a resource of general education on the subject matter. Every effort has been made to ensure the accuracy of the information it contains; however, there is no guarantee that the information will remain current beyond the date of publication. The information and techniques provided in this book should be used in consultation with qualified medical health professionals and should not be considered a replacement, substitute, or alternative for their guidance, assessment, or treatment. The author and publisher accept no responsibility or liability with respect to any person or entity for loss or damage or any other problem caused or alleged to be caused directly or indirectly by information contained in this book.

Contents

Preface

The changes in the number of people dying, the older average age at death, and the decrease in the number of available caregivers are creating a need for health care providers able to care for the dying person and their family. This primary care team is able to meet this need for the majority of people by integrating hospice and palliative care into caregiving. Palliative care is no longer only the specialist's responsibility. Palliative care is every nurse's responsibility. This is known as "integrating a palliative approach."

> *To integrate a palliative approach is to integrate the principles, practices, and philosophy of hospice and palliative care into the care of people with any life-limiting illness, early in the illness trajectory, across all care settings.*
>
> — Kath Murray

Supporting nurses to integrate a palliative approach into care is crucial to providing excellent care for the dying. These learning activities, which are based on the text *Essentials in Hospice and Palliative Care: A Practical Resource for Every Nurse*, are intended to support every nurse to learn the knowledge, skills, and attitudes for integrating a palliative approach and providing excellent care for the dying.

Understanding the Dying Process

Understanding Your Beliefs and Baggage

1. Reflect on the four different patterns (trajectories) of decline and place them in order of your most preferred to least preferred way of dying. Draw and name each pattern on the "flip chart" below. On the right-hand side of the chart, write two reasons why you placed them in the order you did.

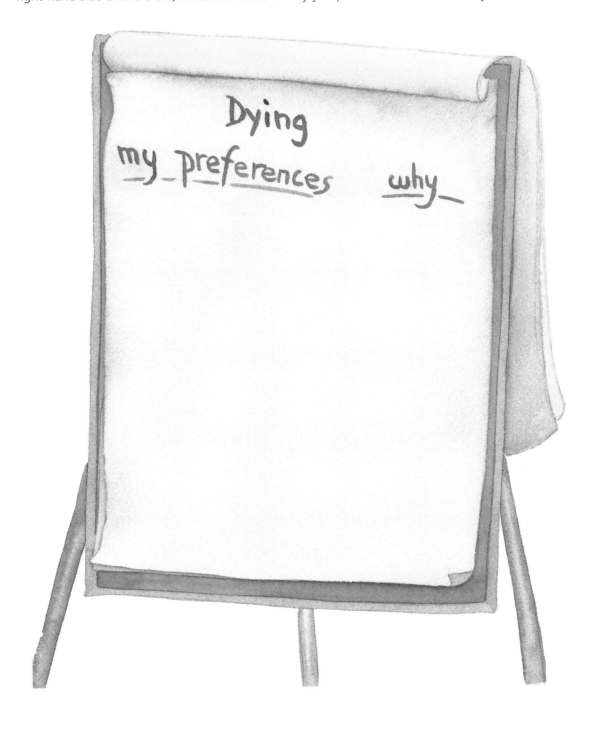

2. Reflect on the trajectories of decline.

   a. Which trajectory would you choose for a loved one? _____

   b. Is the trajectory you chose for your loved one different from the one you chose for yourself? Explain your answer.

   _____

   _____

   _____

   c. Is it harder or easier to imagine and choose a path for someone else? Why? Would you choose more or less aggressive interventions for a loved one?

   _____

   _____

   _____

Solidifying Concepts

3. The 2016 CARES[1] document from the American Association of Colleges of Nursing (AACN) has indicated that new nurses must be able to "identify the dynamic changes in population demographics, health care economics, service delivery, caregiving demands, and financial impact of serious illness on the patient and family that necessitate improved professional preparation for palliative care."

   Choose two areas of dynamic change and explain why these changes will require nurses to be better prepared to provide palliative care.

   _____

   _____

   _____

   _____

   _____

   _____

   _____

   _____

   _____

---

1 Ferrell, B, Malloy P, Mazanec P, Virani R. (2016). *CARES: AACN's New Competencies and Recommendations for Educating Undergraduate Nursing Students to Improve Palliative Care*. Journal of Professional Nursing 32(5), 327–333.

Integrating into Practice

12. Describe something that you can do in your personal or professional life to help reduce the barriers to accessing care that dying people encounter.

_____

_____

_____

_____

13. Describe five actions you can adopt to integrate a palliative approach into your nursing practice.

_____

_____

_____

_____

_____

_____

_____

_____

14. What might a person be experiencing or what challenges might a team be facing that would or should prompt a referral to a hospice and palliative care team specialist?

_____

_____

_____

_____

_____

_____

_____

_____

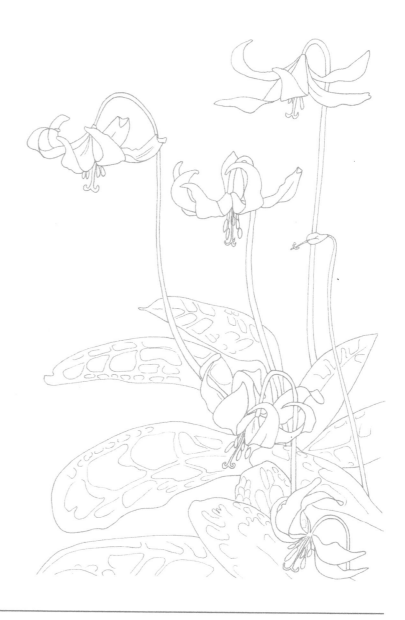

b. Where do your beliefs about a "good" and "bad" death originate (e.g., family, culture, personal experiences, religion, other influences)?

_____

_____

_____

_____

_____

c. Explore with colleagues the similarities and differences in the characteristics of what you consider to be a "good" and "bad" death.

_____

_____

_____

_____

_____

3. Reflect on and write about the value of excellent hospice and palliative care.

_____

_____

_____

_____

_____

_____

_____

_____

_____

_____

_____

_____

_____

_____

_____

4. Circle the faces in the illustration below that reflect some of your feelings about working with people who are dying.

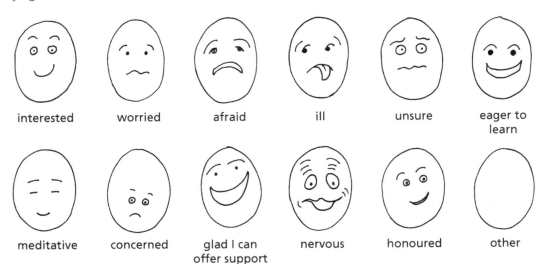

interested   worried   afraid   ill   unsure   eager to learn

meditative   concerned   glad I can offer support   nervous   honoured   other

5. Describe how compassion can be helpful when providing palliative care.

_____

_____

_____

_____

6. Explain how the personal characteristics and ways of being, which Davies and Steele[2] identify as part of best practice, align with the Ethical Responsibilities identified in Canadian Nurses Association Code of Ethics for Registered Nurses, "Part 1-A: Providing safe, compassionate, competent and ethical care.[3]

_____

_____

_____

_____

_____

_____

2   Davies, B., Steele, R., Krueger, G., Albersheim, A., Baird, J., Bifirie, M., Cadell, S., Doane, G., Garga, D., Siden, H., Strahlendorf, C., & Zhao, Y. (2016). "Best practice in provider/parent interaction." *Qualitative Health Research*, 1–15. doi:10.1177/1049732316664712

3   Canadian Nurses Association (2008). "Canadian Nurses Association's Code of Ethics for Registered Nurses. Centennial Edition." https://www.cna-aiic.ca/~/media/cna/page-content/pdf-fr/code-of-ethics-for-registered-nurses.pdf?la=en

12. Write your response to the Dignity Question, "What do I need to know about you as a person to give you the best care possible?" or ask the Dignity Question of a friend or family member.

Reflect on this experience. Share your answer within a small group. Write about the experience. Describe any difficulties. Did any answers surprise you?

_____

_____

_____

_____

_____

_____

_____

_____

_____

_____

_____

_____

_____

_____

_____

_____

_____

_____

_____

_____

_____

_____

_____

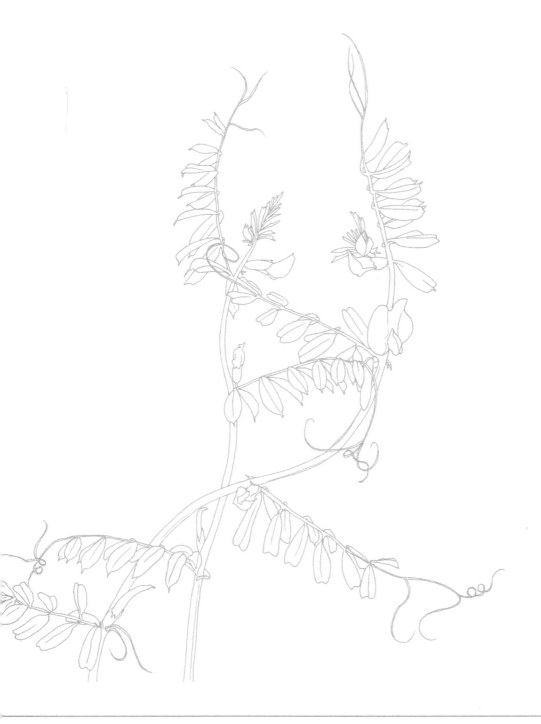

Using Standardized Tools

Solidifying Concepts

1. Describe the rationale for using standardized tools.

   _____

   _____

2. Caregivers in many work settings use the Palliative Performance Scale (PPS) to identify a dying person's current level of functioning and care needs. List five abilities that are measured on the scale.

   a. _____

   b. _____

   c. _____

   d. _____

   e. _____

3. Describe the level of functioning and care needs of a person with a PPS of 40%.

   _____

   _____

   _____

4. Describe the level of functioning and care needs of a person with a PPS of 10%.

   _____

   _____

   _____

5. What does each letter in the mnemonic "OPQRSTUV" of the Symptom Assessment Tool represent?

   _____

   _____

   _____

   _____

   _____

6. Explain why a tool such as the SBAR is important when working with a health care team.

_____

_____

_____

_____

_____

_____

Integrating into Practice

7. Explain the benefits of using a screening tool for integrating a palliative approach into acute and long-term care. Consider the screening tools for integrating a palliative approach (GSF PIG, SPICT, tools for prognosticating one-year mortality). Identify which one is used at your location, or, if one is not currently in use, which one you might consider using.

_____

_____

_____

_____

_____

_____

_____

_____

_____

_____

_____

_____

_____

_____

_____

_____

_____

Sumi Mathew
A483879

Enhancing Physical Comfort

Part 1: Principles of Symptom Management

Understanding Your Beliefs

1. Reflect on your experiences of pain. Reflect on experiences of pain that you have witnessed in your family, friends, and other people you know. Consider your beliefs about pain management. Did you grow up in a home in which family members were comfortable with using medications to manage pain, or do you come from a home in which family members opposed the use of medications for pain management? Write about your responses to these questions.

Solidifying Concepts

2. Complete the crossword puzzle on physical care and comfort measures below.

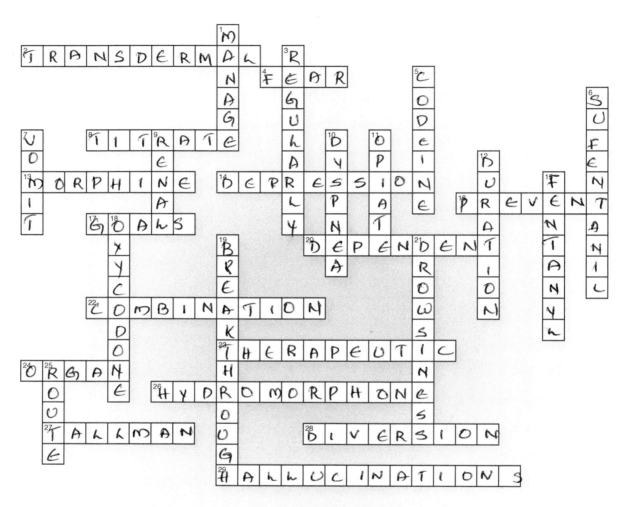

Across

2. Sustained-release opioids may be administered using this method involving a _Transdermal_ patch.

4. Constipation is the number one _fear_ that people express about using opioids.

8. _Titrate_ a medication to the most effective dose.

13. There is no ceiling to the dose of this opioid. _morphine_

14. A person taking opioids who drifts off to sleep during a conversation, may be experiencing respiratory _DEPRESSION_.

16. Breakthrough doses are used to manage breakthrough pain, to help with titration, and to _Prevent_ pain.

17. The principles of symptom management indicate that the focus is on the person's _Goals_ of care.

20. People may fear becoming _Dependent_ on regular doses of opioids.

Sumi Mathew
4483879

22. A ___combination___ of medications may be more effective than a single medication.

23. The range of serum levels of medication that meet the person's goals of care for symptom relief is the ___therapeutic___ window.

24. Checking a person's ___Organ___ function before starting opioids is one step in preventing opioid toxicity.

26. Because it is cleared easily through the kidneys, this is the opioid of choice for people with renal disease. - ___hydromorphone___

27. It is advisable to use this method for writing names of medications when the names are similar and could be confused.

28. When opioid prescriptions or medications make their way to the illegal market, this is called ___diversion___.

29. ___hallucinations___ may indicate opioid toxicity.

Down

1. One principle of symptom management is to ___Manage___ the symptom before it escalates.

3. Managing ongoing symptoms requires medications to be administered around the clock, and ___regularly___.

5. A weak opiate that works well when combined with acetaminophen.- ___codeine___

6. This synthetic opioid is 1000 times more potent than morphine, and is used to treat severe pain.- ___Sufentanil___

7. If a person begins to ___vomit___ partially digested food when they are taking opioids, it may mean that the medication has slowed their GI tract.

9. A person with poor ___renal___ function may not be able to tolerate morphine.

10. Opioids are used for treating pain and ___dyspnea___.

11. The naturally occurring compound found in the resin of poppy plants is an ___opiate___.

12. When using medications, nurses need to be familiar with three parameters of the medication: onset of effect, time to peak effect, and ___duration___ of effect.

15. This opioid is 80 to 100 times more potent than morphine. ___fentanyl___

18. Morphine, 10 mg PO is equivalent to 5 to 7 mg ___Oxycodone___.

19. ___Breakthrough___ pain can occur spontaneously or predictably (e.g., in response to a dressing change).

21. ___drowsiness___ is an initial side effect of starting opioids, and may disappear after a few days.

25. Anticipating ___route___ changes in medications includes arranging for common medications to be kept in stock in a variety of different forms.

(Answer key is on page 89.)

3. Circle the principles of palliation that guide the health care team when managing symptoms.

   a. Focus on the person's goals of care.

   b. Use nonpharmacological comfort measures when possible.

   c. Use medications to manage symptoms only when death is imminent.

   d. Monitor, record, and report the person's responses to medications and other comfort measures

4. Circle the principles that guide the ordering and administration of medications in hospice and palliative care.

   a. The health care team determines the goal for pain relief.

   b. Medications should be given only after pain occurs, not on a regular schedule.

   c. Breakthrough doses are used when a symptom recurs or continues between regularly scheduled doses.

   d. A combination of medications may be necessary to control a symptom and any side effects.

   e. Side effects and fears or concerns about medications should be recorded and reported.

   f. Nonpharmacological comfort measures may help improve comfort.

5. Explain the value of understanding opioid equianalgesia and titration calculations even though nurses are not responsible for ordering opioids.

   -Make sure that the patients need that opiod even though it is prescribed by HCP, the nurses are also accountable if the client experience any promote .
   -educate about the medication usage

6. Why are opioids provided regularly, around the clock?

   Opiods are the drug used as pain reliever which contains chemicals that relaxes the body. it also helps to reduce the incident of giving another pain medication to relieve pain.

7. Identify guidelines to follow when providing nonpharmacological comfort measures.

   - To promote continuity of care by nurse & HCP.
   - Giving comfortable environment .
   - provide measure if its helpful for that — person.
   - Try to use guided imagery or relaxation technique .

8. Discuss the side effects of using opioids and why a person might be concerned about taking opioids.

Alternatively, work in small groups and explore one common side effect associated with taking opioids. Brainstorm ways of communicating with the family when they express concerns about the side effect. Each group can present their findings to the larger group.

_____

_____

_____

_____

_____

_____

_____

_____

_____

9. The family of a dying person is concerned that their loved one is receiving morphine *every four hours!* And sometimes their loved one receives *an extra dose of morphine* before bathing. Discuss, in small groups, how to teach family about the need for medication regularly, around the clock, and the use of break-through doses. You may want to use diagrams to support your discussion.

_____

_____

_____

_____

_____

_____

_____

_____

_____

_____

_____

_____

_____

10. Common myths about opioids can pose significant barriers to opioid use for some people. Identify three common myths and how you might help the person and family to understand the facts.

(a) people that get addicted to opiods can stop
if they try hard enough :- like others opiod misuse
is a long term disease condition. it can alter's one
brain chemistry and its difficult to stop.

(b) only people with addictions are at
risks of overdosing on opiods :- Anyone who use
use opiods are at risk of overdose not anyone
with addiction

11. Angela is currently taking morphine 60 mg po, every 4 hours.

   a. Calculate her 24-hour oral dose of morphine.

   b. Calculate the following equianalgesic doses for Angela:

      i. Morphine long acting po q12h _____

      ii. Morphine subcutaneous q4h _____

12. Michael has advanced esophageal cancer and has been taking morphine 60 mg long acting po q12h. He is no longer able to swallow the tablets. The physician/nurse practitioner has ordered a medication change. Calculate equianalgesic doses of these medications.

   a. Oxycodone rectal q4h _____

   b. Dilaudid subcutaneous q4h _____

13. Daniel rates his pain at 6/10. His current dose of morphine is 30 mg po q4h. He also received four break-through doses (15 mg po morphine) in the past 24 hours. What might be an appropriate new dose for Daniel?

_____

_____

_____

_____

14. The physician has ordered morphine 50 mg po q4h and morphine 5 mg po for a breakthrough dose.

   a. What is the problem with the breakthrough dose? Why?

   _____

   _____

   _____

   b. Calculate the appropriate breakthrough dose (show calculations).

   _____

   _____

   _____

   _____

   _____

   _____

   _____

   _____

   _____

Enhancing Physical Comfort

Part 2: Symptoms

Anorexia and Cachexia

Understanding Your Beliefs

1. Imagine that you look in the mirror and you have lost so much weight that you do not recognize the person who stares back at you. Reflect on and write about your feelings.

    _____

    _____

    _____

    _____

    _____

    _____

    _____

    _____

    _____

2. Describe how the following two experiences might feel different and have different meanings:

    "I have the flu and I am nauseated" versus "I have cancer and I am nauseated."

    _____

    _____

    _____

    _____

    _____

    _____

    _____

    _____

    _____

3. Reflect on the role of food in nurturing your family. Hypothesize and describe reasons why a decreasing appetite could be a difficult symptom for your family to witness.

_____

_____

_____

_____

_____

_____

_____

_____

Solidifying Concepts

4. Describe the similarities and differences between anorexia, cachexia, and anorexia-cachexia syndrome that may occur in a person with life-limiting illnesses.

_____

_____

_____

_____

_____

_____

_____

_____

5. Describe the differences between anorexia-cachexia syndrome and starvation.

_____

_____

_____

_____

_____

Integrating into Practice

6. Family is concerned about their loved one's weight loss. What information would you share to address their concerns and help them to understand the normal decline in appetite and in intake?

_____

_____

_____

_____

_____

_____

_____

_____

_____

_____

7. Discuss nonpharmacological comfort measures for supporting a person who is experiencing anorexia and cachexia.

_____

_____

_____

_____

_____

_____

_____

_____

_____

_____

Changes in Bowel Function

Understanding Your Beliefs

1. Describe your thoughts from the last time you felt constipated or experienced diarrhea. Did you share what you were experiencing with family? Friends? How is sharing information about changes in bowel function different from sharing information when you have a common cold or flu?

    _____

    _____

    _____

    _____

    _____

    _____

    _____

    _____

    _____

    _____

    _____

Solidifying Concepts

2. **a.** List three causes of constipation and provide examples of each.

    _____

    _____

    _____

    _____

    b. What causes diarrhea? What factors may cause this change in bowel function?

    _____

    _____

    _____

    _____

    _____

3. When using the Victoria Bowel Performance Scale to assess a person, it is important to know what is normal stool consistency and frequency for that person. Why?

_____

_____

_____

_____

4. Will it be helpful to increase the intake of dietary fiber in the last weeks or days of a person nearing end of life? Explain your answer.

_____

_____

_____

_____

5. Identify five nonpharmacological comfort measures to implement "in the moment" when a person is experiencing diarrhea.

_____

_____

_____

_____

_____

6. List five pharmacological treatments that can reduce constipation and increase comfort.

_____

_____

_____

_____

_____

_____

_____

_____

Integrating into Practice

7. Consider the case study on page 132 in the text. Describe the information you would share with Mr. Johnson and his family regarding his constipation. What strategies might you recommend to increase his comfort?

_____

_____

_____

_____

_____

_____

_____

_____

_____

_____

_____

_____

_____

_____

_____

_____

_____

_____

_____

Delirium

Understanding Your Beliefs

1. What are your beliefs about delirium? What are your personal or professional experiences with the symptom of delirium?

   _____

   _____

   _____

   _____

   _____

   _____

   _____

   _____

   _____

   _____

2. Why might delirium be frightening to the person or family?

   _____

   _____

   _____

Solidifying Concepts

3. a. What is the definition of delirium?

   _____

   _____

   _____

   b. How would you describe delirium to family?

   _____

   _____

   _____

   _____

4. Identify causes of delirium on the diagram below. Use a highlighter pen to indicate causes that are normal changes in the dying process.

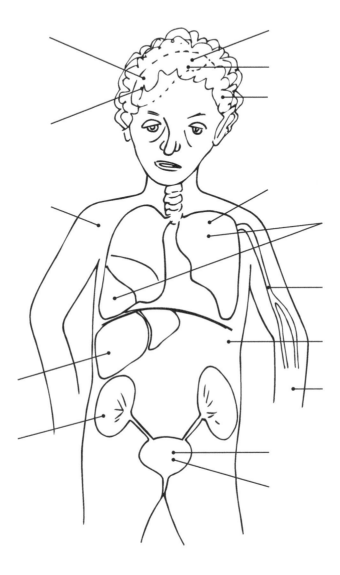

5. What are the differences between dementia and delirium?

_____

_____

_____

6. Delirium is more likely to be reversed if it is _____ _____ , acted on _____ , and if the causes are _____ and can be _____.

Integrating into Practice

7. Case Study

   Marion Beck is a frail 87-year-old woman with moderate dementia. She rates 7, severely frail, on the CSHA Clinical Frailty Scale (she is completely dependent on others for activities of daily living). She has a history of osteoarthritis, back pain, and knee pain. For the past four months, she has taken morphine long acting, 15 mg po q12h.

   In the last several days, she became very agitated, refusing food and resisting care. Marion no longer recognizes health care providers whom she used to know. She is paranoid that someone is coming to get her and has refused medications, saying they are poison.

   a. Explain the potential implications of these changes in her behavior.

   _____

   _____

   _____

   _____

   b. Write notes for a verbal report that you will provide to the physician/nurse practitioner, using the SBAR format.

   _____

   _____

   _____

   _____

   c. Identify nonpharmacological comfort measures you could implement immediately.

   _____

   _____

   _____

   _____

   d. What concerns might the family have about Marion, her condition, and the care that the team provides?

   _____

   _____

   _____

   _____

e. If you identify that Marion is experiencing a delirium, would it be appropriate to investigate the cause? Why or why not?

_____

_____

_____

_____

_____

_____

8. What is the significance of Marion's level of frailty for her prognosis, and how might her frailty affect the decision to investigate or not investigate?

_____

_____

_____

_____

9. In a group, consider Marion's case and discuss the importance of involving the family in decision making and care planning as much as possible.

_____

_____

_____

_____

_____

_____

10. Why might delirium be an especially difficult symptom for families to witness?

_____

_____

_____

_____

_____

_____

Dyspnea

Understanding Your Beliefs

1. Complete the dyspnea exercise described in the video "Dyspnea—the Feeling of Breathlessness" or as described in the activity on page 145 of the text. In the space below, answer the reflection questions listed in the activity in the text.

_____

_____

_____

_____

_____

_____

_____

_____

_____

_____

_____

_____

_____

_____

_____

_____

_____

_____

_____

_____

_____

_____

2. Answer the questions in the first Ethics Touchstone on page 154 in the text.

_____

_____

_____

_____

_____

_____

_____

_____

_____

_____

_____

_____

_____

_____

Solidifying Concepts

3. Define dyspnea.

_____

_____

_____

_____

_____

_____

4. Identify in the diagram below the causes of dyspnea.

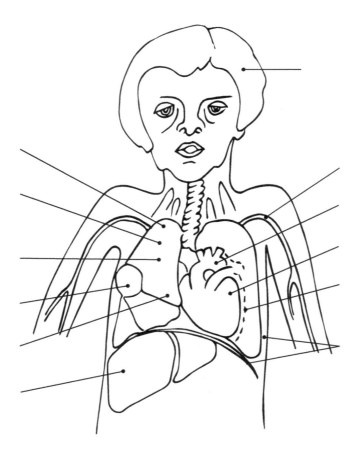

5. The words a person uses to describe their dyspnea may provide insight about the cause of their dyspnea. Identify the three causes of dyspnea that research has linked to the terms "air hunger," "work," and "tightness?"

_____

_____

_____

_____

6. What words or phrases might trigger you to assess a person for dyspnea?

_____

_____

_____

7. Does a person experiencing dyspnea always experience low levels of blood oxygen saturation? Explain your answer.

_____

_____

_____

_____

8. Does every person report their dyspnea? Why or why not?

_____

_____

_____

_____

9. Which tools are recommended for screening, assessing, and monitoring dyspnea?

_____

_____

_____

_____

_____

10. What investigations might be considered when a person has dyspnea? Create a list and include the reasons for each investigation.

_____

_____

_____

_____

_____

11. Describe four strategies for preventing dyspnea.

_____

_____

_____

_____

Integrating into Practice

12. Case Study

Jason Maher is 52 years old and has cancer of the esophagus that has spread to his liver. On arrival, you notice that Jason is very short of breath. He acknowledges that he is short of breath and that it is quite uncomfortable, and rates his discomfort at 7/10. He appears anxious but does not like to complain. In the past, lorazepam was not effective in decreasing the sensation of dyspnea. Currently bronchodilators are not effectively relieving the symptom of dyspnea, and diuretics have not seemed to affect his difficulty with breathing.

a. What nonpharmacological comfort measures might you use to help Jason be more comfortable in the moment?

_____

_____

_____

_____

_____

_____

b. Using the Symptom Assessment Tool Adapted for Dyspnea, what questions might you ask to assess Jason's dyspnea?

_____

_____

_____

_____

_____

_____

_____

_____

c. What questions could you ask to help you to understand Jason's subjective experience of dyspnea?

_____

_____

_____

_____

d. List physical behaviors that you might observe in a person experiencing dyspnea that would be helpful in completing your assessment.

_____

_____

_____

_____

_____

_____

e. Use the SBAR tool to summarize the information from the dyspnea assessment and prepare to communicate with a physician/nurse practitioner. In pairs, role play the conversation with the physician/ nurse practitioner.

13. In a two-person role play between a nurse and a person experiencing an acute episode of dyspnea, practice integrating nonpharmacological comfort measures. Switch the roles so that each person plays the part of the person with dyspnea and the nurse.

Write reflectively about this experience. Reflect on whether the comfort measures worked equally well for both people in the role play.

_____

_____

_____

_____

_____

_____

_____

_____

14. Why is it important to treat a person's dyspnea even though it cannot be measured?

_____

_____

_____

_____

_____

_____

15. Why are opioids helpful in relieving dyspnea?

_____

_____

_____

16. Why are the opioid orders different for the two case studies on pages 152 and 153 in the text?

_____

_____

_____

_____

_____

17. What strategies can nurses implement to support a person or family once the person's dyspnea has settled?

_____

_____

_____

_____

_____

18. What other medications might be helpful for managing dyspnea?

_____

_____

_____

_____

_____

19. Case Study

Barbara is 79 years of age, has end-stage cardiac disease and COPD, and has ongoing shortness of breath (SOB) with activity. In the past month, her SOB has increased with activity. She experienced sudden difficulty with breathing last night, and today she is having difficulty with breathing after eating and when she talks (she often pauses when speaking). Barbara's mobility is limited to transferring her to the commode. She has difficulty rating her dyspnea but suggests it is at 6/10. Her fatigue and feelings of weakness over past weeks have been increasing. Pulse oximetry was not taken.

Observations: *Edema: +3 legs up to knees. Uses auxiliary muscles for breathing and gasps when SOB. Resp. rate 30/min, pulse 100 per minute. Less alert. Periods of confusion in past few days. Skin cool, clammy, diaphoretic. Changing condition, no solid food intake for 24 hours, NPO, mouth care only today.*

a. Discuss comfort measures that might be helpful to implement right away.

b. When Barbara's family asks, "Would oxygen would be helpful?" how might you respond? What information do you need to answer this question?

c. When Barbara is congested, the family asks if suctioning secretions from her mouth would be helpful. What is your response? Explain your answer.

d. What medications could be helpful for Barbara and why?

e. Describe the principles for using opioids in managing dyspnea.

_____

_____

_____

_____

_____

_____

f. If you asked the Surprise Question about Barbara, what might your answer be? Explain.

_____

_____

_____

_____

_____

_____

_____

_____

20. Working with a colleague, coach a person in the Huffing/Coughing technique. In the large group, debrief about this exercise.

_____

_____

_____

_____

_____

_____

_____

_____

_____

_____

_____

Nausea and Vomiting

Understanding Your Beliefs

1. Describe your feelings about nausea and vomiting. Describe your personal and professional experiences with nausea and vomiting.

_____

_____

_____

_____

_____

_____

_____

_____

_____

_____

_____

_____

_____

2. Describe nonpharmacological comfort measures that you find helpful when you feel nauseated or are vomiting. Are these measures similar to or different from those that other people you know use? (Discuss with colleagues.)

_____

_____

_____

_____

_____

_____

_____

_____

_____

_____

Solidifying Concepts

3. Identify on the diagram below the causes of nausea and vomiting.

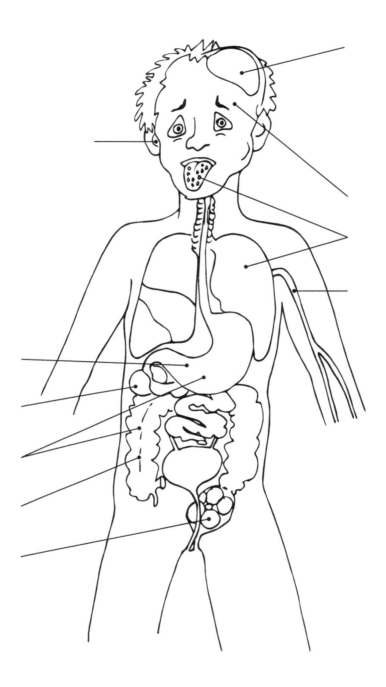

4. How might you explain the common causes of nausea and vomiting to the dying person or the family?

_____

_____

_____

_____

_____

_____

_____

_____

_____

5. Nausea and vomiting are complex symptoms. List some tips that can help you to identify specific causes?

_____

_____

_____

_____

_____

_____

_____

_____

6. What are the steps to managing nausea and vomiting? Why might a person need to continue medications after their nausea or vomiting have settled?

_____

_____

_____

_____

_____

_____

_____

7. Explain why different types of medications may be needed to manage nausea and vomiting resulting from different causes.

_____

_____

_____

_____

_____

_____

_____

8. When might it be appropriate not to rehydrate a person who is dehydrated?

_____

_____

_____

_____

_____

_____

_____

Pain

Understanding Your Beliefs

1. Reflect on a time when you experienced pain. What are your feelings and beliefs about pain?

    _____

    _____

    _____

    _____

    _____

    _____

    _____

    _____

    _____

    _____

    _____

    _____

2. What are your beliefs about the use of medications to manage pain?

    _____

    _____

    _____

    _____

    _____

    _____

    _____

    _____

    _____

    _____

    _____

    _____

3. What are two comfort measures that help you when you are experiencing pain?

_____

_____

_____

_____

_____

4. What comfort measures do you like to offer when someone is in pain?

_____

_____

_____

_____

_____

Solidifying Concepts

5. Define pain.

_____

_____

_____

_____

6. Define total pain.

_____

_____

_____

_____

7. Among people who are dying, pain is a prevalent symptom. What populations are at high risk for untreated pain?

_____

_____

_____

_____

8. Label causes of pain on the body diagram below. Use a colored highlighter and a legend to identify causes that have a common origin.

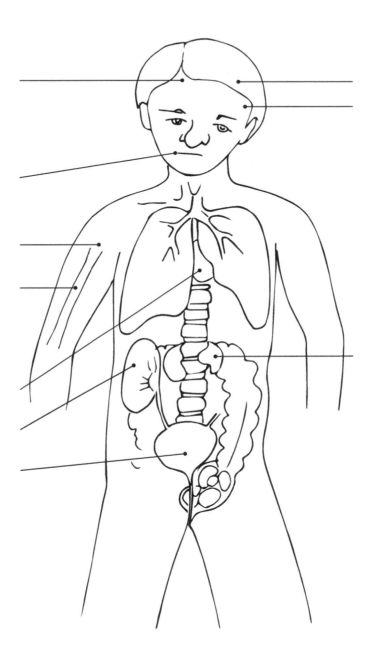

9. Describe nociceptive pain and give examples of different types of nociceptive pain.

_____

_____

_____

_____

10. Describe neuropathic pain and give examples of different types of neuropathic pain.

_____

_____

_____

_____

11. Identify tools used for assessing pain in cognitively intact and cognitively impaired persons.

_____

_____

12. Does the score from the PAINAD scale indicate the severity of pain? Why or why not?

_____

_____

13. How might a body map be useful for assessing pain?

_____

_____

_____

14. List the six categories of behaviors that might indicate pain, as identified by the American Geriatrics Society.

_____

_____

_____

15. Why is it important to obtain input from the family and other health care providers when assessing for pain in a person with cognitive impairment?

_____

_____

_____

16. When would you use the PAINAD scale, the NOPAIN tool, and the Facial Grimace and Behaviour Assessment Tool? How are these tools different in what they assess?

_____

_____

_____

_____

_____

17. What factors determine whether to investigate for causes of pain?

_____

_____

_____

_____

18. Fill in the table below with information about adjuvants.

	Type of adjuvant	How it reduces pain	Example of drug
1.			
2.			
3.			
4.			
5.			
6.			

Integrating into Practice

19. Identify five nonpharmacological comfort measures for preventing pain.

_____

_____

_____

_____

20. In pairs or small groups, practice positioning and then turning in small increments a person experiencing pain, as you would when providing care through the night. What was challenging about this exercise?

_____

_____

_____

_____

_____

_____

21. In pairs or small groups, complete a role play in which one person plays the role of a person experiencing a specific type of pain. Practice selecting and implementing nonpharmacological comfort measures to respond to a person who is in pain. Switch roles so that each person can role play the nurse.

Write reflectively after completing the role plays. How did you decide which comfort measures to use? Was the comfort measure helpful? What do you need to know to implement nonpharmacological comfort measures?

_____

_____

_____

_____

_____

_____

_____

_____

_____

_____

22. In the large group, discuss the following questions. Use the space below to make notes on the discussion.

   a. When should pain be assessed?

   b. Who is responsible for assessing pain?

   c. What behaviors might indicate that a person is experiencing pain?

   d. Discuss different sources of pain and how each is described.

   _____

   _____

   _____

   _____

   _____

   _____

   _____

   _____

   _____

23. Case Study

   Mr. Kirk has lived on the long-term care unit for two years. He is 85 years old and has osteoporosis and a history of multiple fractures. Mr. Kirk is cognitively able and alert, but is very frail and slow moving.

   Today when you help him get up he is hesitant to move and gets out of bed very carefully. When you comment on his slow movements and his apparent stiffness, he says that he is in pain and that he can hardly move because his back is so sore. He says he did not sleep much last night. He is willing to get up to sit in the chair by the bed but does not want to go to the dining room for breakfast. He is very worried about his back.

   a. In a role play, work in pairs to assess Mr. Kirk for pain, using appropriate tools. Prepare an SBAR to communicate the findings of your assessment and your request/recommendation to the physician/nurse practitioner.

   _____

   _____

   _____

   _____

   _____

   _____

b. Write the report you would give to the physician/nurse practitioner to communicate the changes in Mr. Kirk's condition.

_____

_____

_____

_____

_____

_____

_____

_____

_____

_____

_____

_____

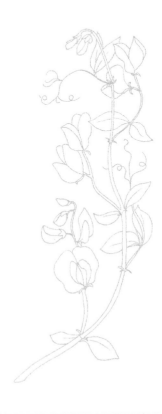

4. What does the word "spirituality" mean to you? What has influenced this understanding (e.g., culture, family, religious teachings, personal experiences)?

_____

_____

_____

_____

_____

_____

_____

_____

_____

_____

5. If the word "spirituality" does not resonate with you, describe the beliefs and ideologies that provide you with strength, hope, connection, meaning, and purpose.

_____

_____

_____

_____

_____

_____

_____

_____

_____

_____

_____

_____

6. Describe your beliefs regarding talking with children about dying and death. What do you recall about the beliefs of your parents or caregivers about children and death?

_____

_____

_____

_____

_____

7. This exercise is designed to help you understand the importance of helping people with life-threatening illnesses determine their priorities and maintain their choices.

    a. In the large box on the next page, write down all that is important to you in your life (e.g., people, activities, events, foods).

    b. In the medium-sized box, write about what you would do if you had only three months to live.

    c. In the small circle, write about what you would do if you had only three days to live.

        Note: If you are feeling vulnerable and think that this exercise will be too much for you, work with a colleague or the instructor to adapt this activity to meet your needs. If this exercise triggers strong responses, consider debriefing with a colleague or the instructor.

        Now think about your responses to the exercise and do some reflective writing guided by the questions below:

    d. What were your feelings as you wrote in the large box? The medium box? The small circle? What thoughts do you associate with these feelings?

        _____

        _____

        _____

        _____

    e. Write about your decision-making process on what to write in the shapes. Did you change your mind? How did you make a final decision?

        _____

        _____

        _____

        _____

        _____

f. How would you feel if you were not able to do what you wrote in the circle?

_____

_____

_____

_____

_____

_____

a

b

c

Solidifying Concepts

8. In the table below, identify the psychosocial changes that commonly accompany the Palliative Performance Scale (PPS) transitions shown in the left-hand column. In the right-hand column, list ways that a nurse can provide support at each transition.

PPS transition	Psychosocial changes	Support nurse can provide
100%–90%		
80%–70%		
60%–50%		
40%–30%		
20%–10%		
0%		

9. Explain why a person might experience multiple losses when living with chronic life-limiting illness. How might integrating a palliative approach provide the best support?

_____

_____

_____

_____

10. Define the terms "loss" and "grief." How might understanding these terms help people experiencing losses and grief?

_____

_____

_____

_____

21. List and explain the rationale behind the principles for supporting a child whose loved one is dying.

_____

_____

_____

_____

_____

_____

_____

_____

_____

_____

_____

22. Describe three concerns children are likely to have when a parent is dying.

_____

_____

_____

_____

_____

_____

_____

_____

_____

_____

_____

_____

_____

Integrating into Practice

23. Complete this multiple losses exercise to learn about your personal responses to loss.

a. On each of six pieces of paper, write down one activity that you enjoy (writing lightly with the pencil will decrease the chance of the writing being legible from the reverse side of the paper when it is turned writing side down). Lay the papers writing side down on the table in front of you. Shuffle them around such that you no longer know which is which. Line them up in a row.

b. Turn over the middle two pieces of paper and imagine that because of declining health you are no longer able to do these activities. What is your immediate response to having these two activities removed from your life? What do you feel? What do you think? Resist the urge to change an activity that you lost to a different one. This exercise is designed to help you imagine the multiple losses that dying people experience. Write your thoughts about this action.

_____

_____

_____

_____

_____

_____

_____

c. Now imagine it is two weeks later and the doctor tells you that you should no longer do two more of the activities. What do you feel about these new losses? Do you feel better knowing that you still have two activities left?

_____

_____

_____

_____

_____

_____

_____

Caring in the Last Days and Hours

Understanding Your Beliefs

1. Reflect on and write about your feelings with respect to providing care for a person in their last days and hours, and at the time of death. Compare this reflection to the feelings you identified in response to question 4 in the learning activities for Chapter 3 about working with people who are dying. Your feelings today may be similar to those you identified before or may have changed.

    _____

    _____

    _____

    _____

    _____

    _____

    _____

    _____

    _____

    _____

    _____

    _____

2. Write reflectively on how you feel about caring for a person's body after death. If you feel uncomfortable, who might you ask to mentor you to increase your comfort? You may want to ask for additional opportunities at work to gain experience providing this kind of care.

    _____

    _____

    _____

    _____

    _____

    _____

    _____

    _____

    _____

    _____

Solidifying Concepts

3. Sometimes the person or family is not willing to talk about death. What strategies might a nurse employ in such a situation to communicate information about dying and death?

_____

_____

_____

_____

_____

_____

4. Explain why it is important to arrange for ongoing support, 24/7, for the family of a dying person. What questions might the family be asking?

_____

_____

_____

_____

_____

_____

_____

_____

_____

_____

5. Define the term "palliative sedation therapy" and describe how is it different from physician assisted dying?

_____

_____

_____

_____

_____

_____

_____

_____

_____

6. Use the information in Chapter 7: Caring in the Last Days and Hours to fill in the following table.

Physical changes in the last days and hours	Supporting the dying person	Supporting the family
Decreased physical strength and increased drowsiness		
Reduced intake and difficulty swallowing		
Delirium and confusion		
Agitation or restlessness		
Unresponsiveness		
Irregular breathing		
Congested breathing		
Changes in skin colour and temperature		
Dry eyes		
Other changes		

7. Describe ways that a nurse could respond supportively when a person might be experiencing final gifts.

_____

_____

_____

_____

_____

_____

8. What physical signs indicate that the person has died?

_____

_____

_____

_____

9. When a person has died and a do not resuscitate (DNR) form has been signed, what can a nurse do?

_____

_____

_____

_____

_____

10. Identify three ways to show respect and support for people whose cultural traditions and spiritual practices are different from yours.

_____

_____

_____

_____

_____

_____

_____

Integrating into Practice

11. Consider the list of questions commonly asked by family when a loved one is dying (see page 232 in the text). Identify questions that you might have difficulty answering. Work with a partner to develop answers that you can use to help become more comfortable in communicating this information.

_____

_____

_____

_____

_____

_____

_____

_____

_____

_____

12. Use the Psychosocial Assessment Form on pages 82 to 88 in the text. With a colleague, participate in a role play to familiarize yourself with asking these questions to obtain information. Were any of the questions difficult to ask? Reflect and consider your beliefs that may have made the question difficult. How might you reframe your beliefs to enable you to become comfortable completing a psychosocial assessment?

_____

_____

_____

_____

_____

_____

_____

_____

_____

_____

13. Compassion is very important to the dying person and family. Why? How might nurses ensure they are providing care with compassion?

_____

_____

_____

_____

_____

_____

_____

_____

14. In the group, discuss the procedure of caring for the body after death in accordance with the guidelines at your location. Ask questions if you are unclear about any aspects or are uncertain about what to do.

_____

_____

_____

_____

_____

_____

_____

_____

_____

3. Review the information about compassion fatigue in Chapter 7 of the text.

   a. Write freely for five minutes about compassion fatigue.

   _____
   _____
   _____
   _____
   _____
   _____
   _____
   _____
   _____
   _____
   _____
   _____
   _____
   _____
   _____
   _____
   _____
   _____
   _____
   _____
   _____
   _____
   _____
   _____
   _____
   _____
   _____
   _____

b. Review the chart on pages 256 and 257 in the text. Circle below which zone you are in.

Green   Yellow   Red

c. Respond to the reflection questions in the table that relate to the zone you are in.

_____

_____

_____

_____

_____

_____

_____

_____

_____

_____

_____

_____

_____

_____

_____

_____

_____

_____

_____

_____

_____

_____

_____

_____

_____

_____

4. Self-care can be integrated into your working life. The following story describes a difficult death and follow up care. The nurse and PSW did a few key things that helped the family and probably helped themselves to feel more at peace with the death, and satisfied with the care they provided. Identify what the nurse and PSW did that benefited the family and themselves.

The death had been difficult. In the end, the man tried to climb out of bed and died in the process. The family was exhausted, sobbing, and distressed.

At the family's request, the nurse provided tea and helped them settle in the living room. Then the nurse and the PSW went to care for the man who had died. They entered the room, shut the door, took some deep breaths, and opened the window to let fresh air fill the room. They played his music quietly.

The nurse began by asking the PSW what she knew about the man who had died. The PSW began to tell the story of a wonderful man, his fascinating life, and how he was much loved by his devoted family. Together the nurse and the PSW talked back and forth while they gently washed the body, changed the sheets, cleaned, and tidied the room, and threw out the garbage. Then they stood at the bedside, hand in hand, in a moment of silence.

The nurse, PSW and the family picked a few of the man's much-loved flowers from his garden and gathered together around the bedside. In this space, the family reminisced and shared memories and stories. The ritual of caregiving brought order out of chaos and prepared a space for the family to come together to honor their loved one.

5. Which self-care strategies might you be interested in trying in the future?

_____

_____

_____

_____

_____

_____

_____

_____

_____

_____

_____

_____

_____

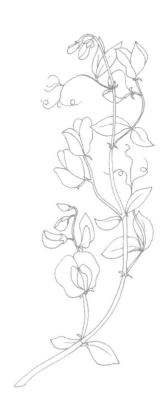

Appendix

Answers to physical care and comfort measures puzzle, page 22

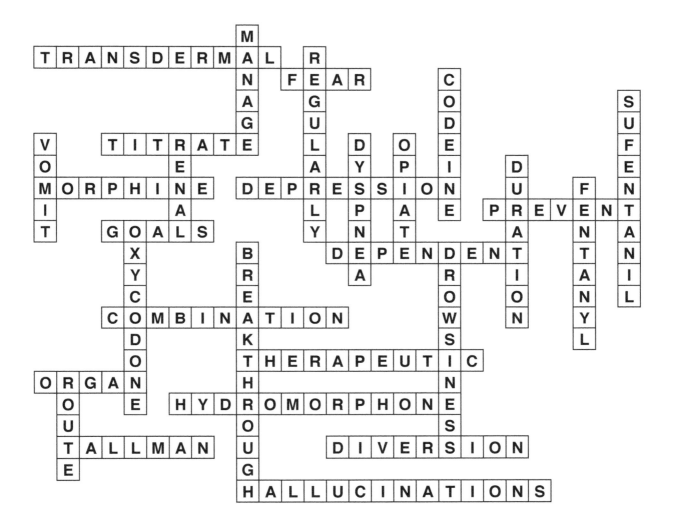

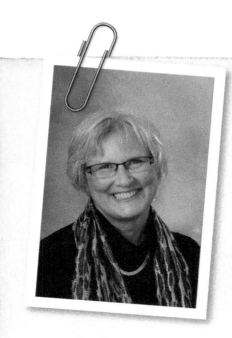

Please feel free to email me your reflections. I so appreciate receiving feedback and stories.

May you feel more comfortable, be more competent, and provide excellent care for the dying and their families. And may your work enrich and bless your life.

Warm regards,

Kath Murray